THE ESSENTIAL PLANT BASED DIET COOKBOOK

The Most complete cookbook guide with 50 recipes to lose weight fast and reset metabolism. Lose up to 7 pounds in 7 days with simple and clear instructions.

Ursa Males

TABLE OF CONTENTS

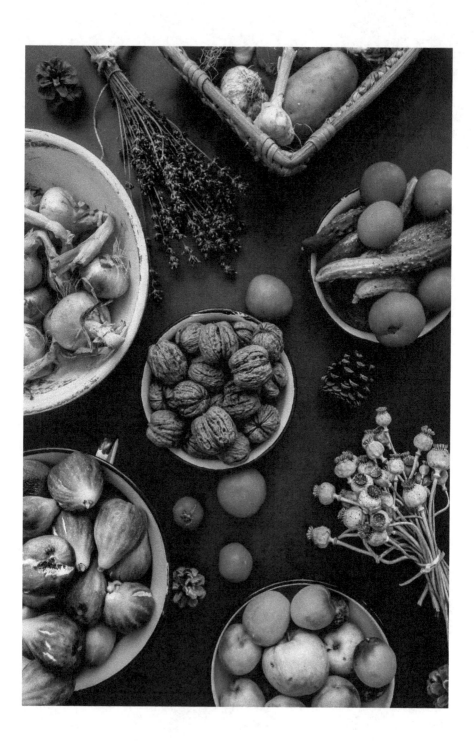

BREAKFAST

1. Tropi-Kale Breeze

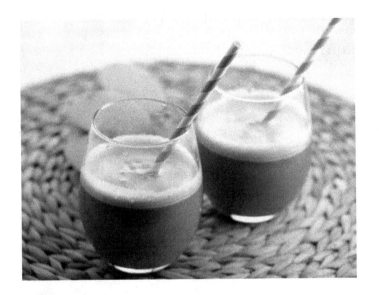

Preparation time: 5 minutes

Cooking time: 0 minutes

Servings: 3-4

Ingredients:

- 1 cup chopped pineapple (frozen or fresh)
- 1 cup chopped mango (frozen or fresh)
- ½ to 1 cup chopped kale
- ½ avocado
- ½ cup of coconut milk

- 1 cup water or coconut water
- 1 teaspoon matcha green tea powder (optional)

Directions:

1. Purée everything in a blender until smooth, adding more water (or coconut milk) if needed.

Nutrition: Calories: 566 Fat: 36g Carbs: 66g Protein: 8g

2. **Hydration Station**

Preparation time: 5 minutes

Cooking time: 0 minutes

Servings: 3-4

Ingredients:

- 1 banana
- 1 orange, peeled and sectioned, or 1 cup pure orange juice
- 1 cup strawberries (frozen or fresh)
- 1 cup chopped cucumber
- ½ cup of coconut water
- 1 cup of water
- ½ cup ice
- Bonus boosters (optional):
- 1 cup chopped spinach
- ¼ cup fresh mint, chopped

Directions:

1. Purée everything in a blender until smooth, adding more water if needed.

2. Add bonus boosters, as desired. Purée until blended.

Nutrition: Calories: 320 Fat: 3g Carbs: 76g Protein: 6g

3. <u>Mango Madness</u>

Preparation time: 5 minutes

Cooking time: 0 minutes

Servings: 3-4

Ingredients:

- 1 banana
- 1 cup chopped mango (frozen or fresh)
- 1 cup chopped peach (frozen or fresh)
- 1 cup strawberries
- 1 carrot, peeled and chopped (optional)
- 1 cup of water

Directions:

1. Purée everything in a blender until smooth, adding more water if needed.

Nutrition: Calories: 376 Fat: 2g Carbs: 95g Protein: 5g

4. <u>Chocolate PB Smoothie</u>

Preparation time: 5 minutes

Cooking time: 0 minutes

Servings: 3-4

Ingredients:

- 1 banana
- ¼ cup rolled oats or 1 scoop plant protein powder
- 1 tablespoon flaxseed or chia seeds
- 1 tablespoon unsweetened cocoa powder
- 1 tablespoon peanut butter, or almond or sunflower seed butter
- 1 tablespoon maple syrup (optional)
- 1 cup alfalfa sprouts or spinach, chopped (optional)
- ½ cup non-dairy milk (optional)
- 1 cup of water
- Bonus boosters (optional):
- 1 teaspoon maca powder
- 1 teaspoon cocoa nibs

Directions:

1. Purée everything in a blender until smooth, adding more water (or non-dairy milk) if needed.

2. Add bonus boosters, as desired. Purée until blended.

Nutrition: Calories: 474 Fat: 16g Carbs: 79g Protein: 13g

5. Pink Panther Smoothie

Preparation time: 5 minutes

Cooking time: 0 minutes

Servings: 3

Ingredients:

- 1 cup strawberries
- 1 cup chopped melon (any kind)
- 1 cup cranberries or raspberries
- 1 tablespoon chia seeds
- ½ cup coconut milk, or other non-dairy milk
- 1 cup of water
- Bonus boosters (optional):
- 1 teaspoon goji berries
- 2 tablespoons fresh mint, chopped

Directions:

1. Purée everything in a blender until smooth, adding more water (or coconut milk) if needed. Add bonus boosters, as desired. Purée until blended.

Nutrition: Calories: 459 Fat: 30g Carbs: 52g Protein: 8g

6. <u>Banana Nut Smoothie</u>

Preparation time: 5 minutes

Cooking time: 0 minutes

Servings: 2-3

Ingredients:

- 1 banana
- 1 tablespoon almond butter/sunflower seed butter
- ¼ teaspoon ground cinnamon
- Pinch ground nutmeg
- 1 to 2 tablespoons dates or maple syrup
- 1 tablespoon ground flaxseed, or chia, or hemp hearts
- ½ cup non-dairy milk (optional)
- 1 cup of water

Directions:

1. Purée everything in a blender until smooth, adding more water (or non-dairy milk) if needed.

Nutrition: Calories: 343 Fat: 14g Carbs: 55g Protein: 6g

7. __Oatmeal Breakfast Cookies__

Preparation time: 15 minutes

Cooking time: 12 minutes

Servings: 5

Ingredients:

- 1 tablespoon ground flaxseed
- 2 tablespoons almond butter/sunflower seed butter
- 2 tablespoons maple syrup
- 1 banana, mashed
- 1 teaspoon ground cinnamon
- ¼ teaspoon ground nutmeg (optional)
- Pinch sea salt
- ½ cup rolled oats
- ¼ cup raisins, or dark chocolate chips

Directions:

1. Preheat the oven to 350°F. Prepare your large baking sheet lined with parchment paper. Mix the ground flax with just enough water to cover it in a small dish, and leave it to sit.

2. In a large bowl, mix the almond butter and maple syrup until creamy, then add the banana. Add the flax-water mixture.

3. Sift the cinnamon, nutmeg, and salt into a separate medium bowl, then stir into the wet mixture. Add the oats and raisins, and fold in.

4. Form 3 to 4 tablespoons batter into a ball and press lightly to flatten onto the baking sheet. Repeat, spacing the cookies 2 to 3 inches apart.

5. Bake within 12 minutes, or until golden brown. Store the cookies in an airtight container in the fridge, or freeze them for later.

Nutrition: Calories: 192 Fat: 6g Carbs: 34g Protein: 4g

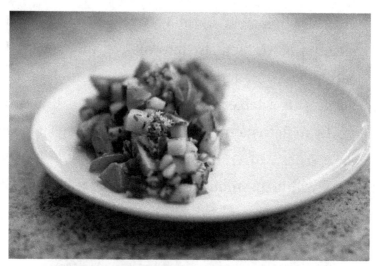

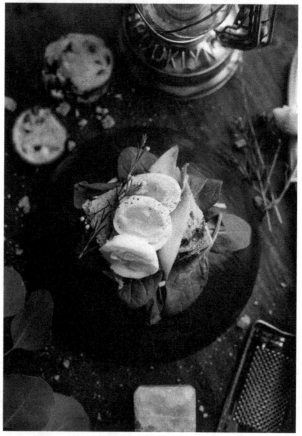

LUNCH

8. Steamed Eggplant with Cashew Dressing

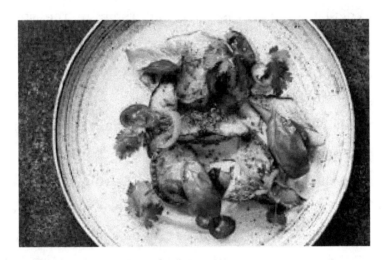

Preparation time: 15 minutes

Cooking time: 0 minutes

Servings: 5

Ingredients:

- 3 small eggplants
- ¼ cup vegan mozzarella cheese
- 1 tbsp. water
- 1 tbsp. soy sauce
- 1 tbsp. chili oil
- 1 tbsp. toasted sesame seeds
- ½ shallot (minced)

- 1 tbsp. dried cilantro

Directions:

1. Fill a large pot (with a steamer on top) halfway with water and put it over medium-high heat. Halve the eggplants lengthwise and put them in the steamer basket once the water is simmering.
2. Steam the eggplant halves for about 15 minutes until they are soft and tender.
3. Meanwhile, add the vegan mozzarella, water, soy sauce, and chili oil to a medium-sized bowl and whisk thoroughly until all ingredients are combined.
4. Once the eggplant halves are cooked, remove them from the heat and arrange them on a medium platter.
5. Drizzle the mozzarella mixture over the eggplant halves and top with the sesame seeds, minced shallot, and cilantro. Serve warm and enjoy!

Nutrition: Calories: 168.5 Carbs: 9.8 g. Fat: 11.5 g. Protein: 4.9 g.

9. Eggplant Chips 'N Dips

Preparation time: 15 minutes

Cooking time: 25-30 minutes

Servings: 12

Ingredients:

- 2 large eggplants
- 1 tsp. salt
- 2 tbsp. olive oil
- 1 garlic clove (minced)
- 1 tbsp. oregano
- 1 tbsp. smoked paprika
- 1 tsp. ground cumin
- Salad:
- 4 cups fresh baby spinach (rinsed and drained)
- ½ cup pickled red cabbage (chopped)
- ½ red onion (finely chopped)
- 1 tbsp. lemon juice
- Dips:
- ½ cup mozzarella cheese
- ½ cup guacamole
- ½ cup Mexican salsa

Directions:

1. Warm oven to 350°F/175°C. Cut the eggplants lengthwise into ¼ inch slices and lay them out in one layer on a baking tray lined with parchment paper.

2. Sprinkle the salt on the layer of eggplant slices and set them aside for about an hour to let the salt dry out the slices. Gently remove excess moisture with paper towels.

3. In a medium-sized bowl, put the olive oil, minced garlic, oregano, smoked paprika, and cumin. Mix thoroughly until everything is combined.

4. Brush each side of the eggplant slices using the spice mixture, making sure all slices are evenly coated.

5. Spread out the eggplant slices in one layer back onto the baking tray, leaving space between each slice.

6. Put the baking tray in your oven and bake for about 25 to 30 minutes, until browned and crispy. Toss all salad fixings in a large bowl, then divide between two medium-sized bowls.

7. Take the baking tray from the oven and let the chips cool for a minute. Put half of the eggplant chips into each bowl and serve with half of each dip. Enjoy!

Nutrition: Calories: 134 Carbs: 6.45 g. Fat: 10.1 g. Protein: 3.3 g.

10. **Mango Lettuce Wraps**

Preparation Time: 10 Minutes

Cooking Time: 10 Minutes

Servings: 4

Ingredients:

- ½ cup Cucumber, seeded & diced
- 1 tbsp. Grapeseed Oil
- ¼ cup Mint Leaves, chopped
- 8 oz. Tempeh, crumbled
- 8 Bibbs Lettuce
- 2 tbsp. Hoisin Sauce
- ¼ cup Cashews, roasted & chopped
- 1 tbsp. Lime Juice
- ¼ cup Mint Leaves, chopped
- ¾ cup Mango, diced

Directions:

1. To begin with, take a large skillet and heat it over medium-high heat. Once the skillet becomes hot, spoon in the oil.

2. Next, stir in the tempeh and sauté them for 4 minutes or until lightly browned. Stir frequently. Then, pour the lime juice and hoisin sauce into the skillet. Mix well.

3. Now, remove the skillet from the heat. Finally, divide the tempeh, mango, roasted cashews, cucumber, and mint between the lettuce leaves. Serve immediately.

Nutrition: Calories: 216 Proteins: 13.4g Carbohydrates: 18.8g Fat: 11.7g

11. <u>Sweet Potato Arugula Salad</u>

Preparation Time: 10 Minutes

Cooking Time: 10 Minutes

Servings: 1 to 2

Ingredients:

- ½ cup Farro, cooked
- 2 cups Arugula
- 2 tbsp. Pumpkin Seeds, toasted
- ½ cup Parsley, fresh & chopped
- ½ cup Black Lentils, cooked
- ½ cup Mint, fresh & stems discarded
- 1 cup Sweet Potatoes, roasted
- ¼ cup Dill, fresh & chopped
- 2 tbsp. of the below dressing
- For dressing:
- 1 tsp. Black Pepper
- 2 tbsp. Olive Oil
- 2 tsp. Pomegranate Molasses
- ¼ cup Grapefruit Juice
- ½ tsp. Salt
- 1 tsp. Maple Syrup

Directions:

1. For making this healthy salad, toss arugula, lentils, herbs, sweet potatoes, and farro in a large mixing bowl.

2. Then, make the dressing by placing together all the ingredients in another small bowl until combined well. Now, spoon the dressing over the salad ingredients and toss them well.

3. Taste for seasoning and spoon in more salt and pepper if needed. Finally, garnish it with the toasted pumpkin seeds.

Nutrition: Calories: 542 Proteins: 20g Carbohydrates: 73g Fat: 21g

12. **Peanut Soup with Veggies**

Preparation Time: 10 Minutes

Cooking Time: 25 Minutes

Servings: 3

Ingredients:

- 2 tbsp. soy sauce
- 1 cup brown rice
- 1 garlic clove, minced
- ½ of 1 red onion, chopped
- 4 tbsp. peanut butter
- 1 carrot, small & chopped
- 3 tbsp. tomato paste
- ½ of 1 courgette, medium & chopped
- 3 cups vegetable broth
- ½ tbsp. ginger, grated
- 2 tbsp. peanuts
- dash of hot sauce

Directions:

1. To begin with, boil the broth in a large saucepan over medium heat. Allow it to boil. In the meantime, cook the rice by following the instructions given in the packet.

2. After that, stir the onion, carrot, and courgette into the saucepan. Mix well. Next, spoon in the ginger and garlic to the mixture.

3. Then, add the peanuts, tomato paste, and peanut butter to the pan. Combine. Taste for seasoning, then put soy sauce to it. Now, allow it to simmer until the rice gets cooked. Serve it hot.

Nutrition: Calories: 488 Proteins: 15g Carbohydrates: 76g Fat: 15g

13. Cauliflower & Chickpeas Casserole

Preparation Time: 10 Minutes

Cooking Time: 60 Minutes

Servings: 4 to 6

Ingredients:

- 3 Garlic cloves, minced
- 2 cups Vegetable Broth
- 1 cup Brown Rice
- ¼ cup Nutritional Yeast
- 1 Celery Rib, sliced finely
- ½ cup Buffalo Hot Sauce
- ½ of 1 Cauliflower Head, medium & chopped
- 1 tsp. Onion Powder
- 2 cups Chickpeas, cooked

Directions:

1. Preheat the oven to 400 F. After that, place onion powder, broth, nutritional yeast, and hot sauce in a medium-sized pot and heat the mixture over medium-high heat.
2. Allow the mixture to boil. In the meantime, spoon the chickpeas to a casserole dish. Then, top it first with the cauliflower pieces, then the celery, and finally the brown rice.

3. When the broth mixture starts to boil, remove it from the heat and spoon in the garlic. Next, pour the mixture over the casserole dish in an even manner.

4. Now, cover the dish with foil and bake it for 55 to 60 minutes in the middle rack. Serve it hot.

Nutrition: Calories: 413 Proteins: 19.3g Carbohydrates: 74.1g Fat: 5.3g

14. Roasted Vegetables and Quinoa Bowls

Preparation time: 10 minutes

Cooking time: 20 minutes

Servings: 4

Ingredients:

- 3 cups cooked quinoa
- For the Broccoli:
- 2 teaspoons minced garlic
- 4 cups broccoli florets
- ½ teaspoon salt
- ¼ teaspoon ground black pepper
- 4 teaspoons olive oil
- For the Chickpeas:
- 4 teaspoons sriracha
- 3 cups cooked chickpeas
- 2 teaspoons olive oil
- 4 teaspoons soy sauce
- For the Roasted Sweet Potatoes:
- 2 teaspoons curry powder
- 2 small sweet potatoes, peeled, ¼-inch thick sliced
- 1/8 teaspoon salt
- 2 teaspoons sriracha
- 2 teaspoons olive oil

- For the Chili-Lime Kale:
- 1/2 of a lime, juiced
- 4 cups chopped kale
- 1/8 teaspoon salt
- 1/8 teaspoon ground black pepper
- 1 teaspoon red chili powder
- 2 teaspoons olive oil

Directions:

1. Switch on the oven, then set it to 400 degrees F and let it preheat.

2. Prepare broccoli florets and for this, take a large bowl, place all of its ingredients in it, toss until well coated, then take a baking sheet lined with parchment paper and spread florets in a one-third portion of the sheet in a row.

3. Add chickpeas into the bowl, add its remaining ingredients, toss until well mixed, and spread them onto the baking sheet next to the broccoli florets.

4. Add sweet potatoes into the bowl, add its remaining ingredients, toss until well mixed, and spread them onto the baking sheet next to the chickpeas.

5. Place the baking sheet containing vegetables and chickpeas into the oven and then bake for 20 minutes until vegetables have turned tender and chickpeas are slightly crispy, turning halfway.

6. Meanwhile, prepare the kale and for this, take a large skillet pan, place it over medium heat, add 1 teaspoon oil and when hot, add kale and cook for 5 minutes until tender.

7. Then season kale with salt, black pepper, and red chili powder, toss until mixed, and continue cooking for 3 minutes, set aside until required.

8. Assemble the bowl and for this, distribute quinoa evenly among four bowls, top evenly with broccoli, chickpeas, sweet potatoes, and kale and then serve.

Nutrition: Cal 415 Fat 17 g Carbohydrates 54 g Protein 16 g

15. **Sweet Potato and Quinoa Bowl**

Preparation time: 5 minutes

Cooking time: 20 minutes

Servings: 4

Ingredients:

- 2 cups quinoa
- 1 cup diced red onion
- 2 cups diced sweet potato
- 1 1/2 cup raisins
- 1 cup sunflower seeds, shelled, unsalted
- 2 cups vegetable broth

Directions:

1. Take a medium pot, place it over high heat, add quinoa, and sweet potatoes, pour in vegetable broth, stir until mixed and bring it to a boil.
2. Then switch heat to medium-low level, cover pot with the lid, and cook for 20 minutes until the quinoa has cooked.
3. Remove the pot from heat, then fluff quinoa by using a fork. Add onion, raisins, and sunflower seeds, stir until mixed and transfer into a large bowl.

4. Let it chill in the refrigerator for 30 minutes and then serve.

Nutrition: Cal 204 Fat 7 g Carbohydrates 31 g Protein 3 g

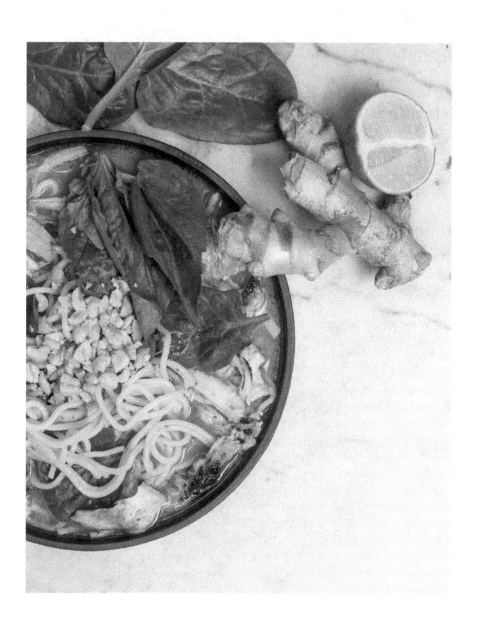

DINNER

16. Thai Red Tofu Curry

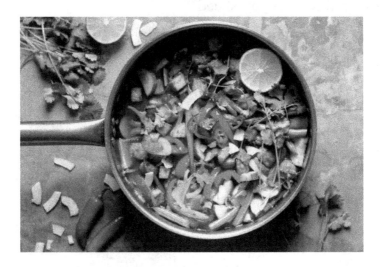

Preparation time: 15 minutes

Cooking time: 22 minutes

Servings: 4

Ingredients:

- 16 oz. Tofu, pressed and cut into ½" cubes
- 4 garlic cloves, minced
- 2 tablespoons sesame oil
- 4 tablespoons soy sauce
- 3 tablespoons rice vinegar
- 1 tablespoon brown sugar

- 1 teaspoon red pepper flakes
- 3 tablespoons corn starch
- 1 yellow onion, minced
- 1 teaspoon ginger, grated
- 1 red bell pepper, sliced
- 1 cup cremini mushrooms, sliced
- 3 tablespoons red curry paste
- 13 oz. Coconut milk
- 1 tablespoon sambal oelek
- 1 lime, zest and juice
- 8 Thai basil leaves, ribboned
- Cooked rice

Directions:

1. Drain and press the tofu within 30 minutes. Mix 1 garlic clove, 3 tablespoons soy sauce, 2 tablespoons sesame oil, 1 tablespoon brown sugar, rice vinegar, red pepper flakes and corn starch in a bowl.

2. Cut tofu into cubes and add to the freezer bag, add the marinade and refrigerate for 30 minutes. Transfer tofu to a bowl and add cornstarch. Mix well.

3. Heat coconut oil in a pan over medium heat. Fry tofu cubes for 2 minutes on each side. Transfer to a bowl.

4. Add ¼ cup water to the pan and bring to a simmer. Add garlic, ginger and minced onion and turn the heat to medium. Cook for 5 minutes. Add mushrooms and

red bell pepper. Add 3 tablespoons red curry paste and mix well.

5. Add coconut milk, lime juice and zest and soy sauce. Mix well and cook for 15 minutes. Serve with rice.

Nutrition: Calories: 307 Carbs: 17g Fat: 19g Protein: 16g

17. **Barbecue Baked Seitan Strips**

Preparation time: 15 minutes

Cooking time: 60 minutes

Servings: 4

Ingredients:

- ½ cup nutritional yeast
- 3 cups vital wheat gluten
- 1 ½ teaspoon smoked paprika
- 1 ½ tablespoon garlic powder
- 1 teaspoon onion powder
- ½ teaspoon dried oregano
- ½ teaspoon dried basil
- 3 ½ cups vegetable broth
- 2 cups vegan barbecue sauce
- 5 tablespoons olive oil
- 5 tablespoons maple syrup
- 3 tablespoons soy sauce
- 1 teaspoon liquid smoke
- 1 teaspoon garlic powder
- 1 ½ teaspoons black pepper

Directions:

1. Preheat the oven to 390f. Mix gluten, yeast, 1 ½ tablespoon garlic powder, 1 teaspoon smoked paprika,

1 teaspoon onion powder, ½ teaspoon black pepper, ½ teaspoon oregano and ½ teaspoon basil in a bowl.

2. Mix 1 cup BBQ sauce, 2 tablespoons maple syrup, 1 ½ cups vegetable broth, 2 tablespoons olive oil and 1 tablespoon soy sauce in a bowl. Add liquid to dry ingredients and mix well. Knead the mixture until the dough is formed. Let rest.

3. Mix the remaining broth, BBQ sauce, maple syrup, olive oil, soy sauce, liquid smoke, black pepper, garlic powder, and smoked paprika in a bowl and mix well to make a marinade.

4. Put your dough on a flat surface and flatten. Add a little oil and roll out to 1" thick and rectangle shape. Add 1 cup marinade to a tray and place dough on top.

5. Cover with the remaining marinade. Bake for 1 hour adds 1 cup broth if it dries in between. Serve and enjoy.

Nutrition: Calories: 533 Carbs: 24g Fat: 25g Protein: 54g

18. Teriyaki Glazed Tofu Steaks

Preparation time: 15 minutes

Cooking time: 10 minutes

Servings: 3

Ingredients:

- 14 oz. Block tofu
- 1 teaspoon garlic, minced
- 1/2 teaspoon ginger, grated
- 1 tablespoon lemon juice
- 4 tablespoons soy sauce
- 2 tablespoons maple syrup
- 1 tablespoon rice vinegar
- 1/4 teaspoon corn starch
- 1/4 teaspoon Dijon mustard
- Oil

Directions:

1. Mix all ingredients except oil and tofu in a bowl to make the sauce. Cut tofu into 1/2" thick slices.
2. Coat a pan with oil and heat over medium-high. Add the tofu steaks. Flip and cook until crust is brown from all sides. Leave last batch in pan and add half of teriyaki sauce.

3. Coat the tofu steaks thoroughly with the sauce and cook for 2 minutes. Repeat with the remaining tofu steaks and sauce. Serve and enjoy.

Nutrition: Calories: 183 Carbs: 8g Fat: 10g Protein: 19g

19. <u>Vegan Chili Sin Carne</u>

Preparation time: 15 minutes

Cooking time: 25 minutes

Servings: 6

Ingredients:

- 3 garlic cloves, minced
- 2 tablespoon olive oil
- 2 celery stalks, chopped
- 1 red onion, sliced
- 2 red peppers, chopped
- 2 carrots, peeled and chopped
- 1 teaspoon chili powder
- 1 teaspoon ground cumin
- 1 lb. canned tomatoes, chopped
- 14 oz 1can red kidney beans, drained & rinsed
- 3 1/2 oz split red lentils
- 14 oz frozen soy mince
- 1 cup vegetable stock
- Salt and pepper, to taste
- Basmati rice, cooked

Directions:

1. Heat olive oil in a pan. Cook carrots, onion, celery, garlic and peppers over medium heat until softened.

Put the chili powder, cumin, salt and pepper and mix well to combine.

2. Add kidney beans. Lentils, chopped tomatoes, vegetable stock and soy mince. Cook for about 25 minutes, stirring often. Serve with basmati rice.

Nutrition: Calories: 563 Carbs: 81g Fat: 10g Protein: 36g

20. Teriyaki Tofu Stir Fry Over Quinoa

Preparation time: 15 minutes

Cooking time: 30 minutes

Servings: 4

Ingredients:

- 1 lb. Asparagus
- 14 oz. Firm tofu
- 2 tablespoon green onions, chopped
- 4 tablespoon tamaris
- 2 teaspoon cooking oil
- 1 tablespoon sesame oil
- 5 garlic cloves, minced
- 1 1/2 tablespoon rice vinegar
- 1/2 tablespoon ginger, grated
- 1/4 cup coconut sugar
- 1/2 cup water
- 2 teaspoon cornstarch
- 4 cups quinoa, cooked

Directions:

1. Cut tofu block in half. Squeeze to remove excess liquid. Cut into 1/2" thick cubes and fry in 1 teaspoon cooking oil on medium-high heat until lightly brown on all sides. Add 1 tablespoon tamari and toss. Set aside.

2. Mix 3 tablespoon tamari, sesame oil, rice vinegar, garlic cloves, ginger, coconut sugar, corn starch and water in a bowl for sauce. Cut asparagus into 2" long pieces and dice other veggies.

3. Heat 1 teaspoon cooking oil in a pan over medium-high heat. Cook diced veggies until crispy. Add in the tofu. Add in the sauce. Lower heat and cook until sauce thicken.

4. Turn off heat and add over the cooked quinoa. Serve and enjoy.

Nutrition: Calories: 190 Carbs: 12g Fat: 14g Protein: 8g

21. Vegan Fall Farro Protein Bowl

Preparation time: 15 minutes

Cooking time: 55 minutes

Servings: 2

Ingredients:

- 1 cup carrots, diced
- 1 cup sweet potatoes, diced
- 15 oz. Can chickpeas, drained and rinsed
- 1 1/2 cups water
- 2 teaspoons cooking oil
- 4 oz. Smoky tempeh strips
- 1/2 cup farro, uncooked
- 2 cups mixed greens
- 2 tablespoon almonds, roasted
- 1/4 cup hummus
- 4 lemon wedges
- Salt and pepper, to taste

Directions:

1. Warm your oven to 375f and prepare a baking sheet.
2. Mix carrots and sweet potatoes with 1 teaspoon cooking oil and salt and pepper in a bowl. Spread on one half of the baking sheet.

3. Mix chickpeas, remaining oil, 1/8 teaspoon black pepper and pinch salt in a bowl. Spread on the second half of the baking sheet.
4. Add tempeh strips on the baking sheet and roast all for 30 minutes. Flip and shuffle everything at half point.
5. Add farro grains, water, and pinch of salt to a pot and place over medium heat. Cover, bring to a boil and reduce the heat and cook for 25 minutes.
6. Divide farro, greens, and roasted tempeh, chickpeas, and potatoes among 4 bowls. Top with wedges, almonds, and hummus. Serve and enjoy.

Nutrition: Calories: 632 Carbs: 99g Fat: 15g Protein: 30g

22. **Black Bean Quinoa Balls and Spiralized Zucchini**

Preparation time: 15 minutes

Cooking time: 55 minutes

Servings: 4

Ingredients:

- 4 zucchinis
- 1/4 cup sesame seeds
- 1 can black beans
- 1/2 cup quinoa
- 2 tablespoon tomato paste
- 1/4 cup oat flour
- 1/2 tablespoon sriracha
- 2 tablespoon nutritional yeast
- 1 teaspoon garlic powder
- 1 1/2 tablespoon herbs, chopped
- 1 tablespoon apple cider vinegar
- 1 cup cherry tomatoes, halved
- 1/2 cup sun-dried tomatoes
- 1 garlic clove
- 2 tablespoon pine nuts, toasted
- 2 tablespoon nutritional yeast
- 1 teaspoon oregano

- A handful basil
- Salt and pepper, to taste

Directions:

1. Add 1 cup water and quinoa to a pot and cook for about 15 minutes. Drain water and let cool. Add black beans to a bowl and mash with a fork.
2. Add sesame seeds, quinoa, oat flour, sriracha, yeast, tomato paste and spices and mix well. Shape the mixture into balls. Place on a lined baking sheet. Bake at 400 f for 40 minutes.
3. Add 1/2 cup cherry tomatoes, sun-dried tomatoes, apple cider vinegar, garlic clove, pine nuts, yeast, basil, oregano and salt and pepper to a blender and blend until creamy to make the sauce.
4. Spiralize zucchinis and add to a bowl. Add tomato sauce and 1/2 cup cherry tomatoes to the bowl and add 5 quinoa balls per serving. Serve and enjoy!

Nutrition: Calories: 382 Carbs: 55g Fat: 12g Protein: 14g

23. **Mongolian Seitan (Vegan Mongolian Beef)**

Preparation time: 15 minutes

Cooking time: 9 minutes

Servings: 6

Ingredients:

- 2 tablespoon + 2 teaspoon vegetable oil
- 3 garlic cloves, minced
- 1/2 teaspoon ginger, minced
- 1/3 teaspoon red pepper flakes
- 1/2 cup soy sauce
- 2 teaspoons corn starch
- 2 tablespoons cold water
- 1/2 cup + 2 tablespoons coconut sugar
- 1 lb. homemade seitan
- Rice, cooked, for serving

Directions:

1. Heat 2 teaspoons vegetable oil in a pan over medium heat. Add garlic and ginger and mix well. Add red pepper flakes after 30 seconds and cook for 1 minute.
2. Add coconut sugar and soy sauce and mix well. Reduce the heat to medium-low and cook for 7 minutes.

3. Mix cornstarch plus water then add to the pan and mix well to combine. Cook for 3 minutes reduce the heat to lowest and simmer.
4. Heat the remaining oil in a skillet over medium-high heat. Add the seitan and cook for 5 minutes.
5. Reduce the heat and add the sauce to the pan. Mix well to coat every seitan piece and cook until all sauce adheres. Remove from heat. Serve with rice.

Nutrition: Calories: 324 Carbs: 33g Fat: 8g Protein: 29g

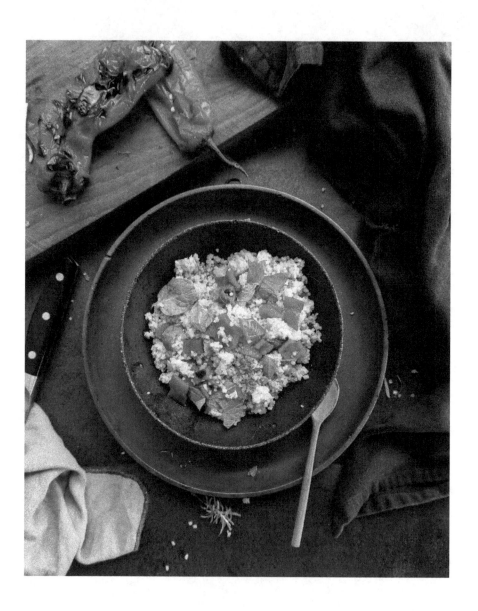

SNACKS

24. Zucchini Sticks

Preparation Time: 10 minutes

Cooking Time: 25 minutes

Servings: 8

Ingredients:

- 2 zucchinis, cut into 3-inch sticks lengthwise
- Salt, to taste
- 2 organic eggs
- ½ cup Parmesan cheese, grated
- ½ cup almonds, grounded
- ½ teaspoon Italian herb seasoning

Directions:

1. In a large colander, place zucchini sticks and sprinkle with salt. Keep aside for about 1 hour to drain. Preheat the oven to 425 degrees F. Line a large baking sheet with parchment paper.
2. Squeeze the zucchini sticks to remove excess liquid. With a paper towel, pat dries the zucchini sticks. In a shallow dish, crack the eggs and beat.

3. In another shallow dish, mix together remaining ingredients. Dip your zucchini sticks in egg then coat with the cheese mixture evenly.

4. Arrange the zucchini sticks into a prepared baking sheet in a single layer. Bake within 25 minutes, turning once halfway through.

Nutrition: Calories: 133 Fat: 9.2g Carbohydrates: 4.5g Protein: 9.4g

25. Strawberry Gazpacho

Preparation time: 15 minutes

Cooking time: 0 minutes

Servings: 4

Ingredients:

- 3 large avocados, peeled, pitted and chopped
- 1/3 cup fresh cilantro leaves
- 3 cups homemade vegetable broth
- 2 tablespoons fresh lemon juice
- 1 teaspoon ground cumin
- ¼ teaspoon cayenne pepper
- Salt, to taste

Directions:

1. In a blender, add all fixings and pulse until smooth. Transfer the gazpacho into a large bowl. Cover and refrigerate to chill completely before serving.

Nutrition: Calories: 227 Fat: 20.4g Carbohydrates: 9g Protein: 4.5g

26. Cauliflower Popcorn

Preparation Time: 10 minutes

Cooking Time: 12 hours

Servings: 2

Ingredients:

- 2 heads of cauliflower
- Spicy Sauce
- ½ cup of filtered water
- ½ teaspoon of turmeric
- 1 cup of dates
- 2-3 tablespoons of nutritional yeast
- ¼ cup of sun-dried tomatoes
- 2 tablespoons of raw tahini
- 1-2 teaspoons of cayenne pepper
- 2 teaspoons of onion powder
- 1 tablespoon of apple cider vinegar
- 2 teaspoons of garlic powder

Directions:

1. Chop the cauliflower into small pieces. Put all the ingredients for the spicy sauce in a blender and create a mixture with a smooth consistency.

2. Coat the cauliflower florets in the sauce. See that each piece is properly covered. Put the spicy florets in a dehydrator tray.

3. Add some salt and your favorite herb if you want. Dehydrate the cauliflower for 12 hours at 115°F. Keep dehydrating until it is crunchy. Enjoy the cauliflower popcorn

Nutrition: Calories: 491 Protein: 19.97 g Fat: 12.84 g Carbohydrates: 86.15 g

27. Quinoa Tabbouleh

Preparation Time: 10 minutes

Cooking Time: 10 minutes

Servings: 6

Ingredients:

- 1 cup of well-rinsed quinoa
- 1 finely minced garlic clove
- ½ teaspoon of kosher salt
- ½ cup of extra virgin olive oil
- 2 tablespoons of fresh lemon juice
- Freshly ground black pepper
- 2 Persian cucumbers, cut into ¼-inch pieces
- 2 thinly sliced scallions
- 1 pint of halved cherry tomatoes
- ½ cup of chopped fresh mint
- 2/3 cup of chopped parsley

Directions:

1. Set a medium saucepan on high heat then boil the quinoa mixed with salt in 1 ¼ cups of water. Set the heat to medium-low, cover the pot, and then simmer everything until the quinoa is tender. The entire process will take 10 minutes. Take off the quinoa from

heat and allow it to stand for 5 minutes. Fluff it with a fork.

2. In a small bowl, put and whisk the garlic with the lemon juice. Add the olive oil gradually. Mix the salt and pepper to taste.

3. On a baking sheet, spread the quinoa and allow it to cool. Shift it to a large bowl and mix ¼ of the dressing.

4. Add the tomatoes, scallions, herbs, and cucumber. Give them a good toss and season everything with pepper and salt. Add the remaining dressing.

Nutrition: Calories: 228 Protein: 9.15 g Fat: 12.09 g Carbohydrates: 20.78 g

28. Hummus Made with Sweet Potato

Preparation Time: 15 minutes

Cooking Time: 55 minutes

Servings: 3-4

Ingredients:

- 2 cups of cooked chickpeas
- 2 medium sweet potatoes
- 3 tablespoons of tahini
- 3 tablespoons of olive oil
- 3 freshly peeled garlic gloves
- Freshly squeezed lemon juice
- Ground sea salt
- ¼ teaspoon of cumin
- Zest from half a lemon
- ½ teaspoon of smoked paprika
- 1 ½ teaspoon of cayenne pepper

Directions:

1. Set the oven to 400°F. Add the sweet potatoes on the middle rack of the oven and bake them for about 45 minutes.

2. Allow the sweet potatoes to cool. Add all the other ingredients in a food processor then blend. After the

sweet potatoes have sufficiently cooled down, use a knife to peel off the skin.

3. Add the sweet potatoes to a blender and blend well with the rest of the ingredients. Once you have a potato mash, sprinkle some sesame seeds and cayenne pepper and serve it!

Nutrition: Calories: 376 Protein: 12.02 g Fat: 20.14 g Carbohydrates: 40.09 g

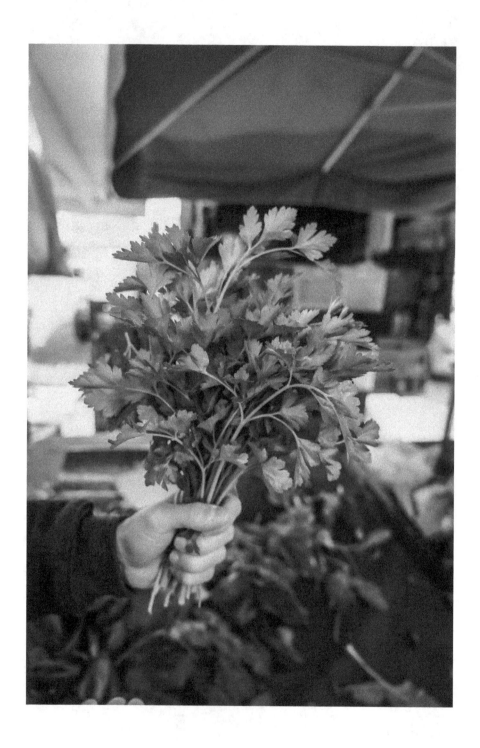

VEGETABLES

29. **Steamed Broccoli with Walnut Pesto**

Preparation Time: 5 minutes

Cooking Time: 10 minutes

Serving: 4

Ingredient:

- 1-pound broccoli florets
- 2 cups chopped fresh basil
- ¼ cup olive oil
- 4 garlic cloves
- ½ cup walnuts
- Pinch of cayenne pepper

Direction:

1. Put the broccoli in a large pot and cover with water. Bring to a simmer over medium-high heat and cook until the broccoli is tender, about 5 minutes.

2. Process basil, olive oil, garlic, walnuts, and cayenne for ten 1-second pulses, scraping down the bowl halfway through processing.

3. Drain and put again to the pan. Toss with the pesto. Serve immediately.

Nutrition: 101 Calories 3g Fiber 5g Protein

30. Roasted Asparagus with Balsamic Reduction

Preparation Time: 10 minutes

Cooking Time: 25 minutes

Serving: 4

Ingredient:

- 1½ pounds asparagus, trimmed
- 2 tablespoons olive oil
- ½ teaspoon sea salt
- ¼ teaspoon freshly ground black pepper
- 1/3 cup balsamic vinegar
- Juice and zest of 1 Meyer lemon

Direction

1. Preheat the oven to 375°F. On a large rimmed baking sheet, throw the asparagus with the olive oil, salt, and pepper and then spread the asparagus out into a single layer. Roast for 23 minutes.
2. While roasting, put the vinegar in a small saucepan and bring it to a boil over medium-high heat. Decrease heat to low and simmer for 8 minutes.

3. When the asparagus is roasted, remove the baking sheet from the oven. Stir lemon juice and zest to coat. Drizzle the balsamic reduction over the top. Serve immediately.

Nutrition: 104 Calories 4g Fiber 8g Protein

SALAD

31. Sweet Potato & Black Bean Protein Salad

Preparation Time: 15 minutes

Cooking Time: 0 minutes

Servings: 2

Ingredients:

- 1 cup dry black beans
- 4 cups of spinach
- 1 medium sweet potato
- 1 cup purple onion, chopped
- 2 tbsp. olive oil
- 2 tbsp. lime juice
- 1 tbsp. minced garlic
- ½ tbsp. chili powder
- ¼ tsp. cayenne
- ¼ cup parsley
- ¼ tsp Salt
- ¼ tsp pepper

Directions:

1. Prepare the black beans according to the method.
2. Preheat the oven to 400°F.

3. Cut the sweet potato into ¼-inch cubes and put these in a medium-sized bowl. Add the onions, 1 tablespoon of olive oil, and salt to taste.

4. Toss the ingredients until the sweet potatoes and onions are completely coated.

5. Transfer the ingredients to a baking sheet lined with parchment paper and spread them out in a single layer.

6. Put the baking sheet in the oven and roast until the sweet potatoes start to turn brown and crispy, around 40 minutes.

7. Meanwhile, combine the remaining olive oil, lime juice, garlic, chili powder, and cayenne thoroughly in a large bowl, until no lumps remain.

8. Remove the sweet potatoes and onions from the oven and transfer them to the large bowl.

9. Add the cooked black beans, parsley, and a pinch of salt.

10. Toss everything until well combined.

11. Then mix in the spinach, and serve in desired portions with additional salt and pepper.

12. Store or enjoy!

Nutrition: Calories 558 Total Fat 16.2g Saturated Fat 2.5g Cholesterol 0mg Sodium 390mg Total Carbohydrate 84g Dietary Fiber 20.4g Total Sugars 8.9g Protein 25.3gVitamin D 0mcg Calcium 220mg Iron 10mg Potassium 2243mg

GRAINS

32. Kale and Sweet Potato Quinoa

Preparation Time: 10 minutes

Cooking Time: 19 minutes

Servings: 4

Ingredients:

- ¼ cup olive oil (optional)
- 1 yellow onion, diced
- 2 tablespoons ground coriander
- 2 tablespoons ground cumin
- 2 tablespoons mustard powder
- 2 tablespoons ground turmeric
- 2 teaspoons ground cinnamon
- 1 large sweet potato, diced
- 1¼ cup uncooked quinoa
- 4 cups water
- 1 bunch kale, rinsed and chopped
- Salt, to taste (optional)
- Freshly ground black pepper, to taste

Directions:

1. In a large pot, heat the oil (if desired) over medium-high heat. Add the onion and sauté for 3 minutes. Stir in the coriander, cumin, mustard powder, turmeric and cinnamon. Cook for about 1 minute, or until fragrant. Add the sweet potatoes and stir until well coated with the spices.

2. Stir in the quinoa and water. Cover with a lid and bring to a boil over high heat, stirring occasionally. Once the liquid is boiling, remove the lid and reduce the heat to medium-low. Simmer for 15 minutes.

3. Once the water is mostly absorbed and the sweet potato is cooked through, stir in the kale. Remove from the heat and cover with a lid. Let sit for 10 to 15 minutes. The residual heat will cook the kale and the quinoa will absorb the remaining water.

4. Taste and season with salt (if desired) and pepper. Divide evenly among 4 meal prep containers and let cool completely before putting on lids and refrigerating.

Nutrition: calories: 457 fat: 16.2g carbs: 67.9g protein: 10.1g fiber: 12.2g

33. Brown Rice with Mushrooms

Preparation Time: 15 minutes

Cooking Time: 20 minutes

Servings: 6 to 8

Ingredients:

- ½ pound (227 g) mushrooms, sliced
- 1 green bell pepper, chopped
- 1 onion, chopped
- 1 bunch scallions, chopped
- 2 cloves garlic, minced
- ½ cup water
- 5 cups cooked brown rice
- 1 (16-ounce / 454-g) can chopped tomatoes
- 1 (4-ounce / 113-g) can chopped green chilies
- 2 teaspoons chili powder
- 1 teaspoon ground cumin

Directions:

1. In a large pot, sauté the mushrooms, green pepper, onion, scallions, and garlic in the water for 10 minutes.
2. Stir in the remaining ingredients. Cook over low heat for about 10 minutes, or until heated through, stirring frequently.

3. Serve immediately.

Nutrition: calories: 185 fat: 2.6g carbs: 34.5g protein: 6.1g fiber: 4.3g

34. Veggie Paella

Preparation Time: 15 minutes

Cooking Time: 52 to 58 minutes

Servings: 4

Ingredients:

- 1 onion, coarsely chopped
- 8 medium mushrooms, sliced
- 2 small zucchinis, cut in half, then sliced ½ inch thick
- 1 leek, rinsed and sliced
- 2 large cloves garlic, crushed
- 1 medium tomato, coarsely chopped
- 3 cups low-sodium vegetable broth
- 1¼ cups long-grain brown rice
- ½ teaspoon crushed saffron threads
- Freshly ground black pepper, to taste
- ½ cup frozen green peas
- ½ cup water
- Chopped fresh parsley, for garnish

Directions:

1. Pour the water in a large wok. Add the onion and sauté for 5 minutes, or until most of the liquid is absorbed.
2. Stir in the mushrooms, zucchini, leek, and garlic, cook for 2 to 3 minutes, or soften slightly.

3. Add the tomato, broth, rice, saffron, and pepper. Bring to a boil. Reduce the heat and simmer, covered, for 30 minutes.

4. Add the peas and continue to cook for another 5 to 10 minutes. Remove from the heat and let rest for 10 minutes to allow any excess moisture to be absorbed.

5. Sprinkle with the parsley before serving.

Nutrition: calories: 418 fat: 3.9g carbs: 83.2gprotein: 12.7gfiber: 9.2g

LEGUMES

35. Beluga Lentil and Vegetable Mélange

Preparation Time: 10 minutes

Cooking Time: 10 minutes

Servings: 4

Ingredients:

- 3 tablespoons olive oil
- 1 onion, minced
- 2 bell peppers, seeded and chopped
- 1 carrot, trimmed and chopped
- 1 parsnip, trimmed and chopped
- 1 teaspoon ginger, minced
- 2 cloves garlic, minced
- Sea salt and ground black pepper, to taste
- 1 large-sized zucchini, diced
- 1 cup tomato sauce
- 1 cup vegetable broth
- 1 ½ cups beluga lentils, soaked overnight and drained
- 2 cups Swiss chard

Directions:

1. In a Dutch oven, heat the olive oil until sizzling. Now, sauté the onion, bell pepper, carrot and parsnip, until they've softened.

2. Add in the ginger and garlic and continue sautéing an additional 30 seconds.

3. Now, add in the salt, black pepper, zucchini, tomato sauce, vegetable broth and lentils; let it simmer for about 20 minutes until everything is thoroughly cooked.

4. Add in the Swiss chard; cover and let it simmer for 5 minutes more. Bon appétit!

Nutrition: Calories: 382; Fat: 9.3g; Carbs: 59g; Protein: 17.2g

36. Mexican Chickpea Taco Bowls

Preparation Time: 10 minutes

Cooking Time: 10 minutes

Servings: 4

Ingredients:

- 2 tablespoons sesame oil
- 1 red onion, chopped
- 1 habanero pepper, minced
- 2 garlic cloves, crushed
- 2 bell peppers, seeded and diced
- Sea salt and ground black pepper
- 1/2 teaspoon Mexican oregano
- 1 teaspoon ground cumin
- 2 ripe tomatoes, pureed
- 1 teaspoon brown sugar
- 16 ounces canned chickpeas, drained
- 4 (8-inch) flour tortillas
- 2 tablespoons fresh coriander, roughly chopped

Directions:

1. In a large skillet, heat the sesame oil over a moderately high heat. Then, sauté the onions for 2 to 3 minutes or until tender.

2. Add in the peppers and garlic and continue to sauté for 1 minute or until fragrant.

3. Add in the spices, tomatoes and brown sugar and bring to a boil. Immediately turn the heat to a simmer, add in the canned chickpeas and let it cook for 8 minutes longer or until heated through.

4. Toast your tortillas and arrange them with the prepared chickpea mixture.

5. Top with fresh coriander and serve immediately. Bon appétit!

Nutrition: Calories: 409; Fat: 13.5g; Carbs: 61.3g; Protein: 13.8g

BREAD & PIZZA

37. __Keto Bread Rolls__

Preparation time: 10 minutes

Cooking time: 20 minutes

Servings: 8

Ingredients:

- 1 1/3 cups almond flour
- 1 1/2 cups shredded mozzarella cheese, part skim
- 2 oz cream cheese, full Fat
- 1 1/2 tablespoon baking powder, aluminum free
- 2 tablespoons coconut flour
- 3 eggs

Directions:

1. Preheat your oven to 350-degree F
2. In a clean bowl, put almond flour, coconut flour and baking powder. Mix well and set it aside.
3. Using a microwave-safe bowl, put the cream cheese and mozzarella in it and microwave for 30 seconds.
4. Remove the bowl, stir and microwave again for 30 seconds. This should go on until the cheese has entirely melted.

5. Using a food processor add the cheese, the eggs and flour mix. Process at high speed for uniformity of the dough. (It is normally sticky.)

6. Knead the dough into a dough ball and separate it into 8 equal pieces. Slightly wet your hands with oil for this step.

7. Roll each piece with your palms to form a ball and place each ball on the baking sheet. (should be 2 inches apart)

8. In a bowl, add the remaining egg and whisk. Brush the egg wash on the rolls.

9. Bake for 20 minutes or until they are golden brown.

Nutrition: Calories 216 Carbohydrates 6 g Fats 16 g Protein 11 g

38. Easy Flatbread Pizza

Preparation time: 10 minutes

Cooking time: 10 minutes

Servings: 3

Ingredients:

- Pita flatbread – 1
- Italian blend seasoning – 1/8 teaspoon.
- Red pepper flakes – 1/8 teaspoon.
- Cherry tomatoes – 1/2 cup, halved
- Mozzarella cheese – 1/2 cup, grated
- Pizza sauce – 3 tablespoons.

Directions:

1. Preheat the oven to 350 F. Spread pizza sauce, cheese, and cherry tomatoes over flatbread.
2. Sprinkle with red pepper flakes and Italian seasoning. Bake in a preheated oven for 10 minutes. Serve.

Nutrition: Calories: 250 Cal, Carbohydrates: 25g, Protein: 5g, Fats: 8g, Fiber: 1g.

SOUP AND STEW

39. **Coconut and Grilled Vegetable Soup**

Preparation Time: 10 Minutes

Cooking Time: 45 Minutes

Servings: 4

Ingredients:

- 2 small red onions cut into wedges
- 2 garlic cloves
- 10 oz. butternut squash, peeled and chopped
- 10 oz. pumpkins, peeled and chopped
- 4 tbsp melted vegan butter
- Salt and black pepper to taste
- 1 cup of water
- 1 cup unsweetened coconut milk
- 1 lime juiced
- ¾ cup vegan mayonnaise
- Toasted pumpkin seeds for garnishing

Directions:

1. Preheat the oven to 400 F.
2. On a baking sheet, spread the onions, garlic, butternut squash, and pumpkins and drizzle half of the butter on

top. Season with salt, black pepper, and rub the seasoning well onto the vegetables. Roast in the oven for 45 minutes or until the vegetables are golden brown and softened.

3. Transfer the vegetables to a pot; add the remaining ingredients except for the pumpkin seeds and using an immersion blender puree the ingredients until smooth.

4. Dish the soup, garnish with the pumpkin seeds and serve warm.

Nutrition: Calories 290 Fat 10 g Protein 30 g Carbohydrates 0 g

40. **Celery Dill Soup**

Preparation Time: 5 Minutes

Cooking Time: 25 Minutes

Servings: 4

Ingredients:

- 2 tbsp coconut oil
- ½ lb celery root, trimmed
- 1 garlic clove
- 1 medium white onion
- ¼ cup fresh dill, roughly chopped
- 1 tsp cumin powder
- ¼ tsp nutmeg powder
- 1 small head cauliflower, cut into florets
- 3½ cups seasoned vegetable stock
- 5 oz. vegan butter
- Juice from 1 lemon
- ¼ cup coconut cream
- Salt and black pepper to taste

Directions:

1. Melt the coconut oil in a large pot and sauté the celery root, garlic, and onion until softened and fragrant, 5 minutes.

2. Stir in the dill, cumin, and nutmeg, and stir-fry for 1 minute. Mix in the cauliflower and vegetable stock. Allow the soup to boil for 15 minutes and turn the heat off.

3. Add the vegan butter and lemon juice, and puree the soup using an immersion blender.

4. Stir in the coconut cream, salt, black pepper, and dish the soup.

5. Serve warm.

Nutrition: Calories 320 Fat 10 g Protein 20 g Carbohydrates 30 g

SAUCES, DRESSINGS & DIP

41. Keto Vegan Ranch Dressing

Preparation time: 5 minutes

Cooking time: 10 minutes

Servings: 3

Ingredients:

- 1 cup vegan mayo

- 1 1/2 cup coconut milk

- 2 scallions

- 2 garlic cloves, peeled

- 1 cup fresh dill

- 1 teaspoon garlic powder

- Salt and pepper to taste

Directions:

1. Add scallion, fresh dill and garlic cloves to a food processor and pulse until finely chopped.

2. Add the rest of the **Ingredients:** and blend until a smooth, creamy consistency is achieved.

3. Makes a great creamy salad dressing. Store in the refrigerator.

Nutrition: Total fat: 11.9g Cholesterol: 0mg Sodium: 50mg Fiber: 4g

42. <u>Cauliflower Hummus</u>

Preparation time: 10 minutes

Cooking time: 20 minutes

Servings: 7

Ingredients:

- 1 large head cauliflower
- 1 tablespoon almond butter
- 1 garlic clove, finely chopped
- 1 tablespoon lemon juice
- 2 teaspoons olive oil
- 1/4 teaspoon cumin
- Salt and pepper to taste

Directions:

1. Cut cauliflower into florets and place in a large microwave-safe bowl. Microwave for 10 minutes on high heat or until completely cooked through.

2. Transfer cauliflower florets to a food processor. Add the rest of the **Ingredients:**

3. Blend until smooth, creamy consistency is reached. Can be stored in the refrigerator in an airtight container for up to 5 days.

4. Makes a great dip for fruits and veggies.

Nutrition: Total fat: 2.7g Cholesterol: 0mg Sodium: 12mg Total carbohydrates: 2.7g

43. __Healthier Guacamole__

Preparation Time: 10 minutes

Cooking Time: 10 minutes

Servings: 4

Ingredients:

- 3/4 cup crumbled tofu
- 2 avocados - peeled and pitted, divided
- 1 teaspoon salt
- 1 teaspoon minced garlic
- 1 pinch cayenne pepper (optional)

Directions:

1. Prepare a food processor then put one avocado and tofu in it then blend well until it becomes smooth. Combine salt, lime juice, and the left avocado in a bowl.
2. Add in the garlic, tomatoes, cilantro, onion, and tofu-avocado mixture. Put in cayenne pepper.
3. Let it chill in the refrigerator for 1 hour to enhance the flavor or you can serve it right away.

Nutrition: calories 534 fat 5 carbs 23 protein 11

APPETIZER

44. <u>Mushrooms with Herbs and White Wine</u>

Preparation Time: 10 minutes

Cooking Time: 15 minutes

Servings: 1

Ingredients

- 1 tbsp Olive oil
- 1 ½ pound Fresh mushrooms
- 1 tsp Italian seasoning
- ¼ cup Dry white wine
- 2 cloves Garlic (minced)
- Salt, as per taste
- Pepper, as per taste
- 2 tbsp Fresh chives (chopped)

Directions:

1. Start by heating the olive oil by placing the nonstick skillet on medium-high flame. Once the oil is heated, toss in the mushrooms. Sprinkle the Italian seasoning and sauté for about 10 minutes. Keep stirring.

2. Pour in the dry white wine and toss in the garlic. Continue to cook for about 3-4 minutes. Season with

pepper and salt. Sprinkle the chives and cook for about a minute. Move into a serving bowl then serve hot.

Nutrition: Calories: 522 Carbs: 27g Fat: 16g Protein: 55g

45. Zucchini Stuffed with Mushrooms and Chickpeas

Preparation Time: 30 minutes

Cooking Time: 30 minutes

Servings: 1

Ingredients:

- 4 zucchinis (halved)
- 1 tbsp olive oil
- 1 onion (chopped)
- 2 cloves garlic (crushed)
- ½ package button mushrooms, sliced (8 ounces)
- 1 tsp ground coriander
- 1 ½ tsp ground cumin
- 1 can chickpeas (15.5 ounce)
- ½ lemon (juiced)
- 2 tbsp fresh parsley (chopped)
- sea salt, as per taste
- ground black pepper, as per taste

Directions:

1. Start by preheating the oven by setting the temperature to 350 degrees Fahrenheit. Take a shallow nonstick baking dish and grease it generously.

2. Use a spoon to scoop out the flesh in the center of zucchini halves. Chop the flesh into Place the zucchini halves onto the greased baking dish.

3. In the meanwhile, take a large nonstick skillet and place it over medium flame. Toss in the onions and sauté for about 5 minutes. Add in the garlic and sauté for 2 more minutes.

4. Now add in the mushrooms and zucchini. Keep stirring and cook for about 5 minutes.

5. Add in the chickpeas, cumin, coriander, parsley, lemon juice, pepper and salt. Mix well to combine.

6. Put the zucchini shells on your baking sheet and fill with the chickpea mixture. Put the baking sheet in your oven and bake for about 40 minutes.

7. Once done, remove from the oven and transfer onto a serving platter. Serve hot!

Nutrition: Calories: 149 Carbs: 10g Fat: 10g Protein: 8g

SMOOTHIES AND JUICES

46. Berry Smoothie

Preparation Time: 5 minutes

Cooking Time: 0 minutes

Servings: 4

Ingredients:

- 1 cup berry mix (strawberries, blueberries, and cranberries)
- 4 Medjool dates, pitted and chopped
- 1½ cups unsweetened almond milk, plus more as needed

Directions:

1. Add all the ingredients in a blender, then process until the mixture is smooth and well mixed.
2. Serve immediately or chill in the refrigerator for an hour before serving.

Nutrition: calories: 473 fat: 4.0g carbs: 103.7g fiber: 9.7g protein: 14.8g

47. **<u>Cranberry and Banana Smoothie</u>**

Preparation Time: 5 minutes

Cooking Time: 0 minutes

Servings: 4

- 1 cup frozen cranberries
- 1 large banana, peeled
- 4 Medjool dates, pitted and chopped
- 1½ cups unsweetened almond milk

Directions:

1. Add all the ingredients in a food processor, then process until the mixture is glossy and well mixed.
2. Serve immediately or chill in the refrigerator for an hour before serving.

Nutrition: calories: 616 fat: 8.0g carbs: 132.8g fiber: 14.6g protein: 15.7g

DESSERTS

48. Apple Cobbler Pie

Preparation Time: 15 minutes

Cooking Time: 25 minutes

Servings: 3

Ingredients:

- 3 cups sliced apples
- 6 cups sliced peaches
- 2 tbsp. arrowroot powder
- ½ cup white sugar
- 1 tsp. cinnamon
- 1 tsp. vanilla
- ½ cup water
- Biscuit Topping Ingredients:
- ½ cup almond flour
- 1 cup gluten-free ground-up oats
- ½ tsp. salt
- 2 tsp. baking powder
- 2 tbsp. white sugar
- 1 tsp. cinnamon
- ½ cup soymilk

- 4 tbsp. vegan butter

Directions:

1. Warm your oven to 400 degrees Fahrenheit. Next, coat the peaches and the apples with the sugar, arrowroot, the cinnamon, the vanilla, and the water in a large bowl.

2. Allow the mixture to boil in a saucepan. After it begins to boil, allow the apples and peaches to simmer for three minutes. Remove the fruit from the heat and add the vanilla.

3. Now, add the dry ingredients together in a small bowl. Cut the biscuit with the vegan butter to create a crumble. Add the almond milk, and cover the fruit with this batter.

4. Bake this mixture for thirty minutes. Serve warm, and enjoy!

Nutrition: Calories: 270 Carbs: 39g Fat: 12g Protein: 2g

49. Pecan Pie Pudding

Preparation time: 5 minutes

Cooking time: 0 minutes

Servings: 1

Ingredients:

- ¾ cup plain full-fat Greek yogurt
- ½ scoop low-carb vanilla protein powder
- 4 tablespoons chopped pecans
- 2 tablespoons sugar-free syrup

Directions:

1. Mix the Greek yogurt plus protein powder in a small bowl until smooth and creamy. Top with the chopped pecans and syrup.

Nutrition: Calories: 381 Fat: 21g Protein: 32g Carbs: 16g

50. <u>Chocolate Avocado Pudding</u>

Preparation time: 5 minutes

Cooking time: 0 minutes

Servings: 1

Ingredients:

- 1 avocado, halved
- 1/3 cup full-fat coconut milk
- 1 teaspoon vanilla extract
- 2 tablespoons unsweetened cocoa powder
- 5 or 6 drops liquid stevia

Directions:

1. Combine all the fixings in a high-powered blender or food processor and blend until smooth. Serve immediately.

Nutrition: Calories: 555 Fat: 47g Protein: 7g Carbs: 26g

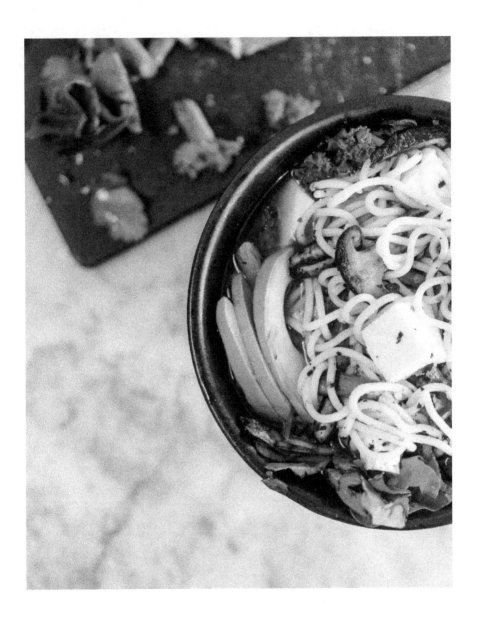